The Best Version Of You

Make the appropriate inquiries of yourself.

Live a more genuine life.

Begin right now.

By

Robert D. Taylor

Introduction

Activities that expand a person's potential and abilities, create human capital, improve employability, improve quality of life, and make ambitions and goals come true are all considered personal development or self-improvement. Personal growth is not restricted to any one stage of a person's life; it can occur throughout their entire lifespan. It is not limited to self-help and can involve both formal and informal acts for the development of others in roles like manager, coach, mentor, guide, or teacher. In the context of institutions, personal development refers to the strategies, plans, instruments, and evaluation frameworks provided to encourage healthy adult development on an individual basis within the company. You'll discover straightforward advice on becoming a better version of yourself in this book. I beg you to pay close attention as you read through the book's chapters and take in these game-changing techniques that have helped me over the years.

TABLE OF CONTENTS

1. The Finest Iteration Of Your Social Self
2. The Finest Iteration Of Your Personal Identity
3. The Healthiest Iteration Of Yourself
4. The Finest Iteration Of Your Academic Self
5. The Finest Iteration Of Your Relationship Self
6. The Finest Iteration Of Your Career Self
7. The Finest Iteration Of Your Spiritual Self

Chapter 1
The Finest Iteration Of Your Social Self

Humans are sociable creatures by nature; we cannot exist in solitude or seclusion. To meet our needs, we rely on one another. We rely on one another to communicate our ideas and emotions. People are social beings. We negotiate through political and economic coalitions, we work in teams, we see responsibility and purpose through religious communion, and our culture shapes our norms. We also live in families. The inherent social traits, inclinations, and actions that define humans are referred to as "man's nature as a social being." It includes interpersonal interactions, the development of relationships, and engagement in social systems. Because of our intrinsic need for community, cooperation, and social connection, humans are regarded as social animals. Humans have always been dependent on one another to survive, to be protected, and to have their emotional and psychological needs met.

what can I do to improve my social skills?

I'm happy you inquired! There's no doubt you can grow or get better at socializing. Here are some broad pointers to get you going:

1. Develop your emotional quotient

Imagine yourself in their position. Consider the circumstances they may be facing and make an effort to comprehend their emotions. Gaining a deeper comprehension of their viewpoint will enable you to reply suitably.

2. Turn your gaze inwards

Be mindful of your feelings, ideas, actions, and stressors. After that, managing them when dealing with others will be simpler.

3. Develop your ability to communicate effectively

To show that you are paying attention, use techniques like open body language and active listening. More constructive encounters are made possible by this.

4. Play it as real as you can

Try behaving like your more gregarious friends, even if it's simply casual conversation. With each attempt, it will get easier.

5. Make more inquiries than statements

You don't need to be shy about speaking up; engage in active listening and pose open-ended inquiries. Individuals enjoy discussing themselves.

6.   Express gratitude

Everybody enjoys a nice complement. Remind someone that their project was excellent or that they did a terrific job at the meeting. Give details.

7.   Be polite

Courtesies have a great impact. Phrases like "thank you" and "please" are simple yet effective methods to soften requests.

8.   Make use of non-verbal cues and open body language

Turn to face the individual you are conversing with. Be mindful of the tone in which you speak. Establish eye contact. To demonstrate that you are present and paying attention, use your body language.

9.   Go through the headlines

Current events are the topic of so many discussions; make an effort to stay up to date so you can contribute.

10.   Refrain from letting your ideas control you

It's acceptable to experience some anxiety, but try not to let it control you. Your thoughts do not make you. You'll feel more at ease in social situations if you take a big breath and try letting them go.

11.   Begin modestly

Spend some time in a coffee shop or work on your conversational abilities with family members to start. You can then gradually go into more social environments. You'll be forming new friendships at your next social event before you know it.

Chapter 2

The Finest Iteration Of Your Social Identity

Measuring your progress requires you to take stock of who you are and where you've come in life. The way you handle other people reveals if you are growing personally or lacking in that area. Here are some suggestions to help you assess yourself.

1. Make individuals feel unique

At every opportunity, empower and encourage others.

2. Find a career you love and give it your all

If you find a job you love, you won't have to work another day in your life.

3. Concentrate on the current task

Make the most out of what you have, where you are now.

4. Give each task due consideration

Each task is a reflection of the individual performing it.

5. Always act morally, even when it is difficult

Don't let your limitations, limit your potential.

6. Assign when you can

When you believe in someone's ability, they will give you their best.

7. Show courage

Try to stretch your boundaries even if you're already highly skilled at what you do.

8. Participate in the fix

Avoid being perceived as someone who is constantly grumbling about anything.

9. Be honest

People should know that they can rely on you to be truthful, even when doing so presents challenges.

10. Along the way, try to help as many people as you can

Turn into someone that others come to for help.

11. Steer clear of gossip at all times

It should go without saying but ignore rumors and gossip

12. Preserve your positive attitude

Happiness is contagious at all times

13. Triple your knowledge to double your income

Keep your knowledge and abilities up to date.

14. Be aware of your feelings

Count to ten when you're upset, and to 100 before you speak.

15. Make tiny daily changes for amazing outcomes

Success is often the result of numerous small everyday efforts.

16. Hone your craft and concentrate on developing your gifts

Steer clear of boredom and pick up a new talent to be competitive.

17. Despite the challenges, be an expert at what you do

When someone tries their hardest, they never fail.

18. Keep your fears at bay

Trust yourself to get through this.

19. Be ready at all times

When preparation meets opportunity, success happens.

20. Seek assistance when you need it

A self-made individual does not exist; you can only succeed in life with the assistance of others.

21. Make plans and achieve them

It's critical to understand your destination, your route there, and the anticipated result.

22. Manifesting your full potential is paramount

Never accept anything lower than your stylish possible outgrowth.

23. Don't stress about getting acknowledgment for completing tasks, you can still negotiate about anything, If you do not watch who gets the credit.

24. Maintain your honesty

Make opinions every day that are in line with your principles.

25. Act as a positive illustration:

Walk the talk and live by your principles.

26. Aspire to standout at everything:

" Do not settle for" good enough."

27. Hold on to your perseverance:

Remaining patient long after others have given up is a crucial element of success.

28. Keep in mind that Leadership is quality you can exhibit anywhere:
Maximize your eventuality in every circumstance.

29. Express thank you and use please at all times because it matters a lot.

30. Respect you get more when you give more

31. Take power:

Accept complete responsibility and transude confidence to complete the task at hand.

32. Decide to give it your all:

It's your determination that will separate the   realizable from the insolvable.

33. Recall that your studies shape who you are barring the bad and emphasizing the positive is pivotal.

34. Remove all conditions:

It feels like you are removing a hundred pounds of cement from your shoulders when you overcome your fears.

35. View lapses as a step up to achievements:

Not trying can be fatal, but failing is noway fatal.

36. Have Credibility:

Make commitments and recognize them.

37. Become an authority:

Maximize the use of your   moxie.

38. Consider the time of others:

Everyone is enthralled. Be brief and direct while trying to get someone's attention.

39. Exercise active harkening:

Make sure you spend at least more important time harkening than talking.

40. Keep your pledges:

Do not break pledges you make.

41. Show excellent cooperation:

Make the utmost of what you can offer.

42. Give up limitations:

Do not allow what you already know to confine you. Aim high and achieve greatness.

43. Solve issues:

When assigned an assignment, complete it efficiently and on schedule.

44. Be open and honest:

People will comprehend your demeanor more completely if you're more open with your information

45. Be kind:

No matter what position you command or how you are feeling, always act with kindness, politeness, and grace toward others.

46. Control your anxiety:

You do not want work- related stress to overcome you, so reduce it at all cost.

47. Be dependable:

Be reliable in your work and constant in who you are.

48. Communicate from the heart sincerity:

It keeps a lot of miscalculations and misconstructions at bay.

49. Work for a cause:

Give everything you do purpose.

50. Stay true to who you are:

Your identity should be reflected in everything you do.

51. Be time conscious:

Until there are no further times to count, we stop counting.

52. Take the arm from within:

You formerly retain all you need to lead a successful life. Well- being is riches. Whatever you put into your body will ultimately manifest. Always flash back to maintain your health by eating well.

Chapter 3

The Healthiest Iteration Of Yourself

You want to constantly radiate your smart health nature, whether you are around family and pals, at work, or at school. You ought to set the same targets for yourself! Because feeling well and robust makes you feel good about yourself, which makes it easier to be a better friend, mate, crew player, and overall individuality. In keeping with that, we have put together a list of course you can do to be the smart interpretation of yourself, both for your own sake and so that you can support the people who count most.

1. Select refections that lift your spirits:
I am apprehensive of how tempting it is to binge on all the genuinely desirable snacks and sweets, similar as deep- fried foods, eyefuls, delicacy, drink, and chips. Still yet, have you supposed about how they make you feel? lassitude, sleepiness, and changes in energy are common responses for multiple of us. This is due to the fact that diets heavy in refined carbs and sugar can raise blood pressure, which in turn causes the body to produce insulin. This combination can beget an inconstancy in your energy strata. A balanced diet that includes whole protein, healthy fats and carbohydrates, and longer- digesting carbohydrates releases sugar into the system more piece by piece and perfectly. Knowing what you are eating by learning to read food markers is one approach to make further amping resolutions.

2.Never give up on knowledge:
It's simple to wax smudged in the day-to-day routine. It's pivotal to commit to being new in order to shake up your routine and widen your skylines. Consider the capacities and interests you retain. Perhaps it's learning a new computer language, instrument, or gift, Perhaps it's reading an important classic literature as you can or seeing every Oscar-winning film on Netflix. Whatever it is, these activities helps keep your health in check.

3. Minimize your consumption of mushy drinks. The main sources of added sugar are mushy drinks including tonics, fruit clouts, and candied teas. Drinking sugar-candied drinks increases the threat of heart complaint

and type-2 diabetes. Beverages with added sugar are especially bad for kiddies since they can induce fatness in kiddies as well as conditions like type 2 diabetes, hypertension, liver complaint, which generally do not manifest until maturity. Better options that are healthier are water with no added sugar, effervescent water, and coffee

4. Consume a lot of fruits and veggies:
Fruits and vegetables are rich sources of antioxidants, vitamins, minerals, and prebiotic fiber, numerous of which have important health benefits. Individuals with advanced fruit and vegetable input live longer and are less likely to suffer from fatness, heart complaint, and other conditions.
5. Cut back on recycled carbohydrates:
Carbs aren't all made equal. The fiber from refined carbohydrates has been considerably recycled out. They have veritably many nutrients and, if consumed in surplus, can be dangerous to your health. Ultra-processed foods are composed of refined carbohydrates similar as white flour, recycled sludge, and added sugars. Eating a diet heavy in refined carbohydrates may increase the threat of weight gain, gluttony, and habitual ailments like heart complaint and type 2 diabetes.

6. Nourish the microorganisms in your stomach:
 Entire health greatly depends on the bacteria in your gut, which are inclusively related to as the gut microbiota. The disturbance of gut vegetation has been connected to a number of long- term ailments, similar as fatness and several digestive issues. Taking probiotic supplements when necessary, eating lots of fiber and consuming fermented foods like yogurt and sauerkraut are all effective strategies to enhance gut health. Especially, fiber provides your gut vegetation with microbiota, acting as a prebiotic and healthy for your guts

7. Exclude redundant abdominal fat:
Visceral fat, or inordinate abdominal fat, is a particularly dangerous form of fat distribution that has been connected to an advanced threat of cardio metabolic ailments like heart complaint and type 2 diabetes. Because of this, your midriff- to- hipsterism rate and midriff size may be far more calculable indexes of health than your weight. You lose belly fat by cutting back on refined carbohydrates, adding your input of protein and fiber, and managing your stress situations, which can lower cortisol, the stress hormone that causes the deposit of belly fat.

8. Steer clear of defined diets:
Diets are infrequently successful in the long run and are generally useless. Actually, one of the stylish pointers of unborn weight gain is once dieting. This is due to the fact that extremely defined diets actually make it harder

to lose weight by lowering your metabolic rate, or the number of calories you burn. Also, they change your hormones that control appetite and malnutrition, making you feel more empty and conceivably driving violent solicitations for foods heavy in fat, calories, and sugar. Consider leading a healthy life as a preference to overeating. Rather than starving your body, concentrate on feeding it. Loss of weight ought to come next as you make the switch to full, nutrient- thick foods, which are by nature more satisfying and lower in calories than recycled foods.

9.Periodically watch your food consumption:
Weighing your food and using a nutrition investigator can be useful tools for certain people to determine how numerous calories they consume. Monitoring can also reveal information on the volume of fiber, protein, and micronutrients you consume. Nevertheless, this tactic can contribute to disordered eating tendencies verily while it may help some people manage their weight Consult a specialist before exercising this tactic.

10. Make liberal use of spices and herbs:
More than ever, we have access to a wide range of sauces and spices these days. They may have several health advantages in addition to adding flavor. For example, the strong anti-inflammatory and antioxidant parcels of gusto and turmeric may help to enhance your general health. You should strive to incorporate a wide variety of sauces and spices into your diet because of their great implicit health advantages.

11. Consume entire eggs:
It's a falsehood that eggs are unhealthy due to their high cholesterol content, despite the ongoing debate concerning eggs and health. The impact of eggs on blood cholesterol situations is negligible for utmost individualities, and they are an excellent reservoir of minerals and protein.

12. Take a moment to meditate:
Your health is negatively impacted by stress. It may have an impact on your blood sugar situations, nutritional preferences, vulnerability to illness, weight, distribution of fat, and other factors. Employing suitable doing mechanisms for your stress is pivotal because of this. One similar system is meditation, which has been shown to be advantageous for reducing stress and enhancing health. Meditation reduces inflammation and LDL(bad)cholesterol.

In summary, your beneficial habits and general heartiness can be greatly enhanced by taking a countless easy measures.
Nevertheless, you should not limit your works to leading a better life to what you put in your mouth. Other rudiments include social relations, sleep, and exercise. Using the forenamed substantiation-grounded advice,

making minor adaptations that can significantly ameliorate your general health is simple.

Chapter 4

The Finest Iteration Of Your Academic Self

You can acquire useful knowledge and critical abilities for self-learning that you can apply to many aspects of your life. To develop into a useful self-learner, you need to experiment with various methods and strategies that can assist you in learning and applying new knowledge. Gaining a lifelong interest in school and studying new topics more easily can be achieved by knowing self-learning tactics.

Here, I will explain self-learning, discuss its advantages, and provide guidelines for using these strategies successfully.

What does self-learning entail::

The process of picking up new information or abilities outside of a formal classroom setting is known as self-learning. It usually entails a variety of methods that can assist you in becoming proficient at learning new things on your own. Self-learning strategies allow individuals to select their study topics, create their research protocols, and define the parameters of their learning process.

You can continue to advance your abilities and acquire technical information outside of the classroom and workplace by engaging in self-learning. For instance, it can assist you in acquiring new skills that can advance your profession, picking up a new interest, or learning a new language.

Getting started on a self-learning process has the following advantages:

1. Build supplementary activities for your profession

Self-learning strategies can help you hone critical job abilities like problem-solving and organizing.

2. Gain greater self-assurance in your abilities: You can inspire yourself to take on new tasks and find solutions to problems by learning how to teach yourself new concepts.

3. Select your learning path

Individuals who learn on their own can choose the methods to employ to acquire new information on their learning preferences, timetables, or learning styles.

4. Learn at your own pace

You may control the speed at which you learn and tailor it to suit your preferences and objectives rather than following a predetermined curriculum.

Chapter 5

The Finest IterationOf Your Relationship Self

To be in a healthy relationship, one must want it more than anything else. It takes a lot of luck in addition to everyone's diligence and hard work. But rather than being a chore, your relationship may also be a lot of fun! As you work through the ideas I'll be sharing with you below, you'll find that you're thinking more carefully about the choices you make, the habits you follow, and eventually your marriage.

Being in a relationship is a fantastic opportunity to grow as a person and see the world from a different angle. Every relationship teaches us something new and alters us internally in both significant and small ways. But it's really simple to lose oneself in a new relationship.

Following these six tips will help you remember to take care of yourself so that you may maintain a connection with yourself even while you are seeing someone else.

How to better myself in a relationship

It's common for our partners to show us so much love that we forget why and how we should love ourselves. Maintaining a connection with yourself inspires you to strive for mental and emotional health, which can strengthen your bond with others.

Of course, there are more rules than just the following six that you should observe. You should take the time to decide what is best for you, taking into account your requirements and the dynamics of your relationship. The following guidance is meant to assist you in coming up with concepts and solutions.

1.Our partners can't always meet our requirements on their own: Everyone needs their mental, bodily, and emotional needs met from time to time. Since they have demands of their own, it would be irrational to expect them to comply. When you take care of yourself, you develop greater emotional intelligence, joy, and self-assurance.

2. Establish boundaries: Even in secure relationships, it's critical to establish boundaries. Contrary to popular belief, defining boundaries doesn't happen until your spouse crosses a certain threshold. Establishing your agency in the relationship and expressing your personal beliefs are the two main goals of setting boundaries.

3. Allow your partner to assist you occasionally. Since your partner cannot read your mind, they will be unable to determine what you need in order to support your personal development. When both partners communicate and uphold their limits to the best of their abilities, the relationship is considered healthy.

4. Strike a balance between taking care of yourself and relying on others: Make an effort to balance helping yourself and your family, friends, or partner while also accepting help in your relationships with yourself. An excessive tendency to tilt one way could be detrimental.

5. Recognize your expectations from a partnership:
Trying too hard to be a lone wolf on your path to self-improvement could cause tunnel vision and block you off to the positive energy your partner can provide. You'll limit your potential and encourage co-dependency if you become unduly dependent on them. Having to always strike a balance between your needs and theirs might also wear your partner out.

6. Motivate your companion to improve:
When couples are constantly bettering themselves while they are together, a love connection is more likely to endure longer, feel better, and more stable. Since it's better to have two emotionally intelligent people than one, if you're focusing on developing yourself, make sure you do everything you can to encourage your partner to do the same. Seeing them flourish can inspire you to look after yourself more, especially during difficult or stressful times.

Altering who you are to fit into a relationship
Your life may change significantly as a result of self-improvement. The problem is, relationships also play a role in it. It might be difficult to discern when you are changing for a love partner and when you are just becoming a better version of yourself.
This is why it is so important to set goals for both the relationship and yourself. In order to stay conscious of your wants, desires, and identity, you must set goals. Allocate some time for introspection so that you may evaluate your own growth following the breakup and figure out how far you still feel you need to go.

How to treat yourself well In a partnership
Self-worth helps you stay anchored in a relationship. Even after you have handed yourself up to someone else and welcomed them into your life, you still need to take certain steps that will help you find, develop, and hold onto the value you possess. In a relationship, whenever you go through any of the following:

1. Self-belief
2. Self-care
3. Believing that the things you do can make people happier
4. Feeling like you're in charge of your life
5. Taking care of your emotional needs;
6. Giving yourself enough time to effectively prepare for challenging situations
7. Getting over miscommunications
8. Having the impression that there is room to grow in your partnership

Chapter 6

The Finest Iteration Of Your Career Self

Why is it crucial to develop personally?

Investing in yourself will enable you to advance in your work and meet professional objectives. Enrolling in a certification program in your field is one way to increase your chances of receiving a promotion. Working on yourself can also help you discover abilities outside of the traditional educational and professional settings. You will benefit in a wide range of work contexts if you have strong hard and soft skills. For instance, you might wish to practice communicating better. After completing that, you could find that you are able to help resolve conflicts between parties through mediation.

How to continuously advance yourself
 1. Read often
Reading regularly is one of the quickest and easiest ways to learn. Regular reading will help you develop a strategic perspective that will advance your career and increase your industry expertise. To increase your knowledge base, look for new sources. Seek writers in other countries and cultures, or read viewpoints that are different from your own. Consider making learning a new language your objective. This will expose you to even more books.
One way to stay up to date is to make a list of the top books, blogs, and publications related to your area and dedicate a specific time each day to reading from it.

2. Take up a new hobby: Despite the fact that your family and job may come first, having a few hobbies is necessary to maintain a healthy work-life balance. Sports, crafts, and other hobbies not only help you learn and grow outside of the office, but they also provide a break from your everyday responsibilities. Think carefully about how you spend your time. Joining a sports team, learning how to make a craft you've never done before, or planning quick excursions are all possible with a few spare hours each week.

3. Enroll in a training session: Although you may be able to master new skills independently, attending a class may provide greater structure to your learning. You can train with an expert to develop hard or soft skills by signing up for an employer-sponsored program after school or during a training session. Sign up for a one-time training session after work to get

started. Once an individual session is over, think about enrolling in a longer class or a multi-session workshop. Carefully consider the topic by determining the exact goals you want to achieve.

4. Identify In-demand skills: If your objective is to develop in your career, identifying the specific abilities needed for advanced tasks may help you become a better version of yourself. Beyond your core competencies, pay attention to new skills that could give you a competitive advantage. Look through trade periodicals to see what skills are most in demand in your industry. Consider signing up for a course to become an authority in these fields and differentiate yourself from the competitors.

5. Consider creating a new schedule: Having a different routine might give you a new perspective on how you spend your time. By reviewing how you spend your day and identifying the times when you are most productive, you may come up with new strategies for making the most of the time you have. For a full week, try rising one hour earlier in order to carve out time for yourself to grow, learn, and improve. Another option is to schedule an hour of reading time before bed or use that hour to start a new hobby during the day.

6. Make a commitment to an exercise regimen: Regular exercise can improve your health, lengthen your life, and improve your quality of life both at work and beyond it. Starting an exercise routine will also help you relax and de-stress, which can boost your output. Consider making a monthly commitment to work out for a few hours each week. Choose an entertaining sport or hobby, and consider working out in the gym with a partner to add some fun to the process. Reward yourself every time you finish a workout. If you miss a workout, strive to get back to your usual schedule as soon as you can to establish a new, healthy habit.

7. Set lofty objectives: A typical day may consist of a number of small chores. Getting to work on time and finishing an assignment are two examples, as is spending dinner with your family and spending meaningful time together. It is even feasible to set longer-term goals, such as saving for a down payment on a house or organizing a summer vacation. If you want to improve yourself, make an effort to think beyond yourself. Consider what you want to do in the next five years, like launching your own company or finding a more rewarding job. Set SMART (specific, measurable, executable, realistic, and time-sensitive) targets after that to develop a plan for accomplishing these objectives.

8.Modify your perspective:
Make an effort to reframe your thoughts. When you shift your perspective, you may find that you have more power over your situation than you

previously believed. By being aware of what you can and cannot control, you can take steps to enhance your quality of life. One possible place to start would be by challenging the status quo and presumptions about your personal circumstances. Think about why you hold the opinions that you do, and push yourself to reconsider the veracity of your convictions.

9. Look for a mentor:
Having someone to lead the way might make self-improvement more enjoyable. Seeking a mentor can help you reach your greatest objectives, regardless of whether you require professional motivation or knowledgeable support. Consider someone you look up to or your dream career in ten years while searching for a mentor. Seek out an expert in your sector with a wealth of knowledge and strong leadership abilities. Think about a mentor who can provide you with the guidance you require to reach your objective.

Chapter 7

The Finest Iteration Of Your Spiritual Self

Spiritual development can be facilitated by regular devotional practices like prayer and church attendance. You can deepen your spiritual connection through engaging in mindfulness practices, contemplating art and the natural world, and producing beautiful things. to develop empathy, transcend oneself, and assist others.

The Four Phases Of Spiritual Development
Reflection:
1.You can grow spiritually by separating yourself from the stressors of daily life and engaging in mindfulness practices. Meditating helps you gain more self-control over your thoughts.
2. You have the choice of doing group or alone meditation.
3. To make your commitment to spiritual contemplation stronger, think about going on a quiet meditation retreat.
4. Take a yoga and meditation session to help you harmonize your mind and body.

Linkage with the surroundings:
1.Go on lengthy, alone outings or take short, sunny walks. Remove your headphones and avoid looking at your phone. Recognize your surroundings. Visit the sea, the mountains, and the desert. Spend some quiet time, unwinding and taking in your surroundings. As you investigate, take a moment to be thankful for your surroundings.
2. Read poems aloud or start a song if you feel moved.
3.To increase your time spent outside, take camping trips.
4. Join those who are interested in spiritual growth for a hike.

Possess an assortment of works of art:
Whether you are on a spiritual journey or belong to a religion tradition that appreciates beauty in art, sacred images and great works of art can help you cultivate a closer relationship with them.
Observe the design, musical selections, and religious artwork found in mosques, churches, temples, and other places of worship.
2. See excellent examples of both religious and secular art by visiting museums.
3. Listen to music that moves you, whether it's traditional or contemporary.

4. Developing a closer relationship with God won't necessarily involve a religious work of art. If an artwork appeals to you, consider it carefully. Try returning to it.

Participate in artistic endeavors:
Creative expression has the power to deepen your spiritual awareness. You can visualize the incomprehensible and become closer to the present by using your creative imagination.
1.Music has long been a traditional way for people of many religious traditions to demonstrate their devotion; it is a typical element of secular spirituality. Learn some hymns or other songs so you can sing on your own or with your family.
2.Dancing is regarded as a form of worship in many cultures. Take a dance class, or just put on some contemplative music and try to dance to it.
3. Any creative activity, including everyday chores like baking, that makes you feel relaxed and centered may be helpful. Give thanks to people who help you. Acknowledge the goodwill you have received from people. Express your gratitude to those who assist you in being the best version of yourself.
4. Sincerely thank people who have helped you. Explain how their actions have benefited you.
5. Keep a gratitude journal in which you write down one or two things every day for which you are grateful.
6. Remember to note the happy feelings you obtain from assisting others. Give them your sincere appreciation for letting you into their lives.

Conclusion

Ultimately, leading a purposeful and happy life is the key to being the best version of yourself in all aspects. Taking care of your health and mind, pursuing your interests and passions, fostering great relationships, putting an emphasis on lifelong learning and development, and giving back to the community are all part of it. The process of personal development, or self-improvement, never stops and finishes only when life does. You must always strive for upward mobility if you want to enhance your living circumstances as well as your physical, mental, and social wellbeing.